Also by Wendy S. Harpham, MD, FACP

Diagnosis: Cancer
After Cancer
When a Parent has Cancer
Becky and the Worry Cup
Happiness in a Storm
Only 10 Seconds to Care

Healing Hope

Through and Beyond Cancer

Wendy S. Harpham, MD, FACP

Illustrations by Emma C. Mathes

Curant House

Healing Hope
Text by Wendy S. Harpham, MD, FACP
Illustrations and design by Emma C. Mathes
Photographs by Benedict F. Voit

Copyright © 2018 Wendy Schlessel Harpham

Contact Curant House for special sales or permission to reproduce selections: *wendyharpham.com/curant-house*
7989 Beltline Road, Suite 305-420, Dallas, Texas 75248

This book is not intended as a substitute for competent medical care. It serves to supplement information provided by your healthcare team.

Library of Congress Control Number: 2017919738

ISBN: 978-0-9997088-1-1

Even in the worst of times, we can strive
to make life the best it can be.

WSH

Table of Contents

You forge and follow your best path with hope. Not just any hope, but hope that helps you think and act in healthy ways.

WSH

Introduction

Aphorisms helped save my life. Those short, powerful statements affected my thoughts and feelings by highlighting truths that helped me deal with the challenges of cancer. My ever-growing repertoire of aphorisms helped me find the courage, fortitude, patience, confidence and hope needed to do all the things that increased my chance of surviving.

I was a busy 36-year-old doctor of internal medicine when diagnosed with a type of cancer with no known cures. Without warning, I had to close my solo practice. My husband and I needed help caring for our 1-, 3-, and 5-year old children. Yet I still had hope. I hoped—we all hoped—the promising new combination of chemotherapy prescribed by my oncologist would cure me. I also hoped my experiences as a patient would make me a better doctor when I resumed patient care and put cancer behind me.

My treatment ordeal ended with my cancer in remission and my hopes soaring. Before my one-year checkup, my cancer recurred. A year later, it recurred again and I retired from clinical medicine. After my ninth course of cancer treatment, my disease went into a remission that has lasted 10 years...and counting.

Everyone tried to encourage me during the rough patches by insisting, "Wendy, be hopeful," as if I could flip on that emotion like a light switch. They didn't seem to understand how difficult it could be to find and maintain hopefulness. It took me years to realize it mattered what I hoped for and that I'd have to create my own path to hope because everyone's path is unique.

Through years of trial and error, I learned which hopes helped me adjust to upsetting news and which hopes helped me make wise decisions. I found hopes that helped me endure tests and treatments, or find patience during recovery, or strengthen my relationship with my healthcare team, or prepare for tomorrow. I conditioned myself to focus on specific hopes that helped me find some happiness, regardless of what was happening medically.

Healthy hope is whatever hope helps you heal.

Even though you will follow your own unique path, common threads run through the tapestry of healing hope after cancer. By "healing hope" I mean hope that helps us through times of uncertainty in healthy ways. Put another way, healing hope helps us get good care and live as fully as possible every day.

Lucky for me, my scientific orientation made it relatively easy to avoid false hope, such as the hope carrot juice could cure lymphoma. I also benefited from the support of an oncology social worker and others with whom I could share whatever I was thinking and feeling without being shut down and told to "be hopeful."

Hope wasn't everything, of course. Logic, trust, discipline and will-to-live also mattered. Hope couldn't help me unless it was based on sound knowledge and I then acted on that knowledge.

In my efforts to survive, hope was only one element—the centerpiece—of my three-step approach to cancer: (1) obtain sound knowledge, (2) nourish healing hope and (3) take effective action. For decades, the knowledge-hope-action approach I named Healthy Survivorship has helped me get good care and live as fully as possible every day. My path to hope continues to be a work-in-progress as I explore, test and practice healing hope. Aphorisms continue to play a major role.

The aphorisms and insights in *Healing Hope* are not solutions to the challenges of cancer; they're tools to give you a leg up in seeing healthy ways to handle your personal health challenges. The aphorisms, supporting text and illustrations are designed to help you think about your own approach to illness—not teach you about me—and to encourage you to begin developing your own personal collection of aphorisms.

Be forewarned: Figuring out what's best for you takes time and effort. *Healing Hope* encourages you to   s l o w   d o w n   and reflect on your thoughts and feelings—especially your hope.

Since the conversations you have with yourself help you define your hopes, *Healing Hope* offers a starting point for healing self-talk. After you close the book, you can continue your hope-based conversations in your head, using whichever ideas, images and aphorisms help you navigate through and beyond cancer.

Before turning to the aphorisms, please read the next section that answers, "What is a Healthy Survivor?" It's okay if you don't like the "survivor" label. It's important we are talking about the same things when I refer to Healthy Survivors and Healthy Survivorship.

When you're ready to read about healing hope, pick a chapter or page that interests you. Read the aphorism. Roll the words around in your mind the way you might finger coins in your pocket to determine their value. Read the supporting text and explore the illustration for additional insights.

Ask yourself what you believe about the idea. Does the aphorism resonate with you? If not, maybe you can maneuver the idea into a personalized aphorism that works better.

What's with the flashlight on the cover? The light of a flashlight serves as my icon for hope. If your experience is anything like mine, making your way through and beyond cancer can feel like walking your life path in the dark. Hope is like a beam of light, helping you see your way, which calms your fears and enables you to move forward as safely and efficiently as possible.

Pursuing unrealistic hope is like shining the light away from your path. That light may calm you, but it doesn't help you move forward—and it may lead you dangerously astray. Also, feeling that hope is out of reach is like seeing a flashlight on a high shelf. You can give up, or you can reach out for help and invest the extra effort needed to benefit from hope. Lastly, even if your hope is accessible and strong now, it may fade if not recharged regularly, like a flashlight in need of new batteries. Nourishing hope takes work.

The power of healing hope changed my life for the better. Today I'm experiencing something I did not expect after my second recurrence: growing old. Did my aphorism-inspired hope cure my cancer? No. Healing hope motivated me to take steps every day to increase my chance of surviving long-term. Healing hope helped me wait when there was nothing I could do to affect the desired outcome. Now, while living with aftereffects of past treatments, healing hope continues to help me get good care and live as fully as possible.

Even if new treatments had not been developed in time for me or my cancer had not responded well to treatments that usually worked, I would have benefited from healing hope. That hope would have guided and supported my efforts to make wise decisions. Healing hope would have motivated me to live as joyfully as possible in whatever time I had.

Healthy Survivorship is an art: the art of living with healing hope through and beyond cancer. These aphorisms have been a gift to me. Now I'm passing them along to you with hope they help you forge and follow the best path for you today, tomorrow and every single day.

With hope,

Wendy

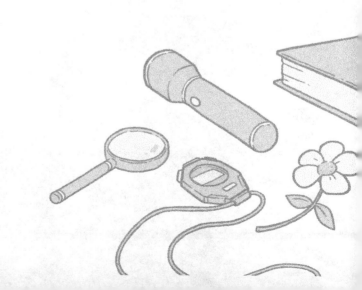

What is a Healthy Survivor?

Many people hate the label "survivor." But we can't escape the fact that cancer patients today are referred to as "survivors" in the professional literatures and in most articles and books for patients. That was not the case when I was diagnosed in 1990. Back then, people with cancer were called "cancer victims."

Lucky for me, a newsletter from the National Coalition for Cancer Survivorship introduced me to "survivor"—the novel concept that would become the norm: "From the time of discovery and for the balance of life, an individual diagnosed with cancer is a survivor."

Without hesitation I adopted the label.

> *"From the time of discovery and for the balance of life, an*
> *individual diagnosed with cancer is a survivor."*
> National Coalition for Cancer Survivorship (1986)

During the months of chemotherapy, my identification as a survivor became problematic. You see, useful labels foster confidence and mobilize us to take effective action. "Survivor" did nothing to encourage me to meet the challenges of my illness. I was a survivor no matter what I thought, felt, said or did. Consider this: You are a survivor whether receiving treatments from a team of top-notch oncologists or swigging snake oil ordered from a website.

You are a survivor whether reveling in gratitude for each day or withdrawing from friends and family due to uncontrolled pain or fear of recurrence. For me, being just a survivor wasn't enough.

I wanted to be a ...(blank)... survivor.

To help me fill in the blank, I asked myself: "Which word describes the type of survivor I aspire to be?" I kept looking for an adjective to describe a person who tackles problems well, namely in healthy ways that promote the desired outcome.

Lo and behold, my question contained my answer: *healthy*. Just as we talk about healthy lifestyles, healthy relationships and healthy financial planning, we can talk about healthy survivorship.

For clarity, in 1992 I defined a Healthy Survivor as a patient who (1) gets good care and (2) lives as fully as possible.

These two criteria inspire excellence without demanding perfection. They do so seamlessly over time as new challenges arise and the ability to respond in healthy ways evolves.

The beauty of this term is that you can be a Healthy Survivor no matter how sick you are or how grim the prognosis. Because Healthy Survivorship is not defined by the biology of your tumor or by your medical outcome. Healthy Survivorship is determined by the quality of your care and by how you live.

> *"A survivor who gets good care and lives as fully as possible is a Healthy Survivor."*
> Wendy S. Harpham, MD (1992)

At times, the pursuit of Healthy Survivorship may feel complicated and demanding. You have to navigate a complex—and, in certain ways, not particularly healing— medical system. You may face unavoidable pain, unwanted change and unanticipated loss. Any of these can lead to a distressing sense of vulnerability and uncertainty, along with grief.

Happiness can seem impossible. It's not.

Each time you act on sound knowledge and realistic hope in healthy ways, you help set the stage for happiness despite illness and, sometimes, because of it. This is the promise of Healthy Survivorship.

Chapter 1:
Knowledge

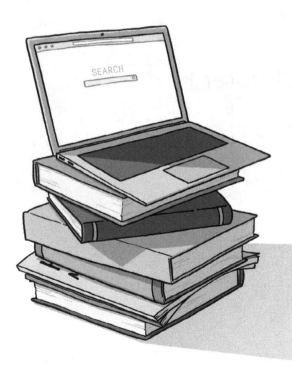

...about KNOWLEDGE

Healthy Survivors learn at least the minimum information about their condition needed to get good care. Considering the explosion of medical information available on the internet, doing so should be as easy as pie. It's not.

Normal fear and sadness can cloud your thinking. The barrage of facts and theories about disease—only some of which are accurate—often causes confusion. Second opinions may cause conflict. And nobody likes learning about possible (or likely) future problems.

When facing medical challenges, knowledge is power—including knowledge about how to obtain sound knowledge. May the aphorisms in this chapter help you overcome obstacles to obtaining the knowledge you need to heal.

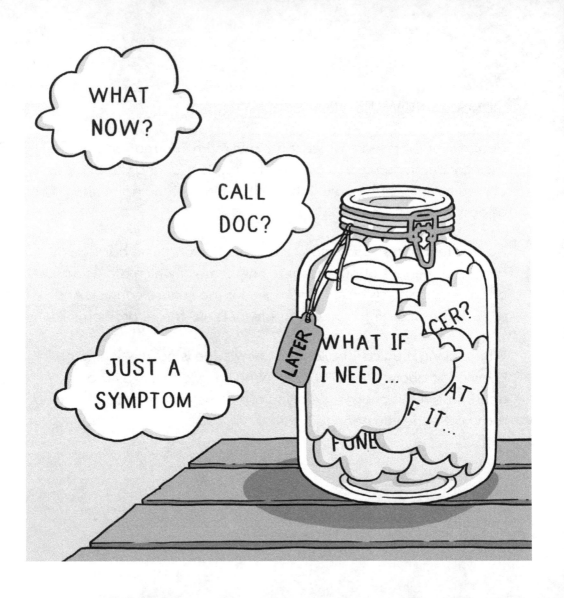

A Cough is Just a Cough

New or increasing symptoms naturally trigger fear:
"It must be cancer."

Stop! This is the wrong time to draw conclusions. Other conditions—including minor problems—can cause the same symptoms. Instead of worrying about what my symptoms might mean, I must act. My job is to notify my doctors: "I have these symptoms. What now?"

Until doctors confirm the cause, I just have symptoms. Not a diagnosis. I must stay in the moment and rein in my imagination. How? By remembering: A pain is just a pain—not a cancer pain. A cough is just a cough.

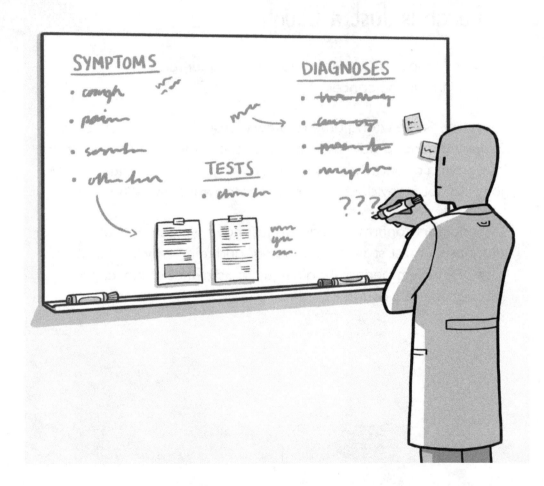

Reporting Symptoms is Not Complaining

I hate complaining to my doctors. Focusing on my discomforts makes me feel worse about my situation. What if my doctors think I'm a whiner?

Here's the thing: For me to receive good care, I must report symptoms. If I keep my symptoms a secret from my doctors, I might as well blindfold and handcuff them. Doctors who don't know about my symptoms can't make timely diagnoses or adjust my medications properly. Worst of all, I might suffer unnecessarily. That would upset everyone–and be miserable for me.

When I talk about my symptoms, I'm not complaining. I'm reporting vital information.

Doctor visits are not social visits.

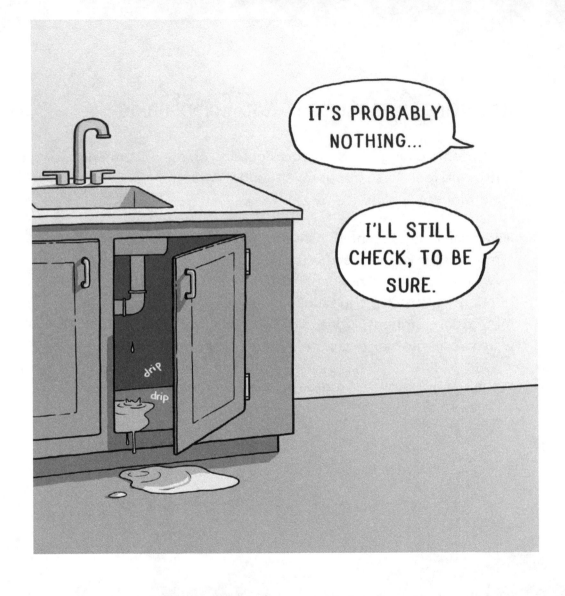

Ignorance is Not Bliss...
When Missing Windows of Opportunity

Learning about potential medical problems upsets me. Since I may never develop a single one, why learn—and worry—about them?

Here's why: So I never look back with regret, saying "(sigh) I wish I knew then what I know now."

Choosing to avoid upsetting topics today means taking the risk of suffering unnecessarily tomorrow. As a Healthy Survivor, I'd rather accept temporary distress now to gain the power to minimize problems that are preventable or treatable.

Ignorance is not bliss when missing windows of opportunity to improve the outcome.

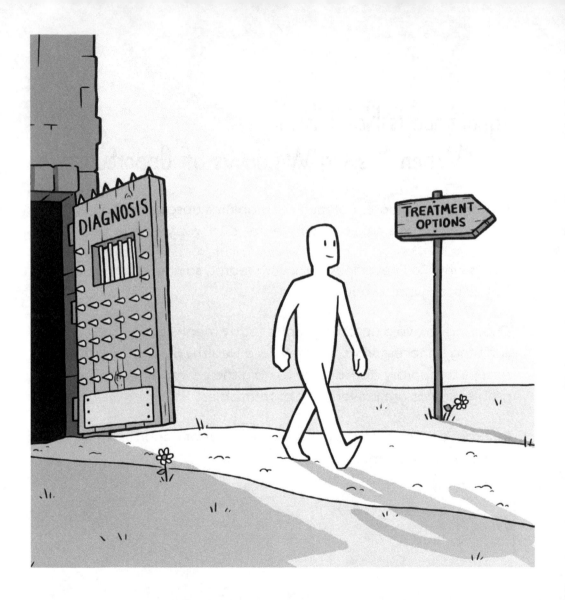

The Diagnosis Sets Us Free...
Even if It Hurts When We Learn It

Until I find out what is causing this new symptom, I'm trapped by fear and anxiety.

If I notify my doctors of my symptom and their evaluation uncovers an easily fixable problem—Yay!—then the truth sets me free. But what if tests reveal some awful problem? Then the truth drags me down into the nerve-racking world of more tests and treatments. Is that free?

Yes. If some problem is brewing, I cannot benefit from treatment and support until after we determine what's wrong. The diagnosis sets me free, even if it hurts when I learn it.

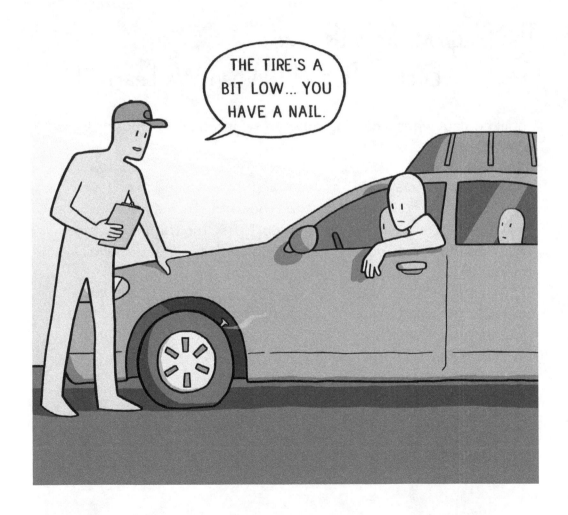

The Best News is Accurate News

Everyone keeps saying, "I hope you get good news."

Hoping for good news is natural, but it doesn't help me. My hope won't change the test results. If I get what I'm hoping for—good news—but the tests missed a problem, then "good news" only delays the diagnosis, which delays treatments.

Whenever I undergo evaluation, more than I hope for good news, I hope for the news that can help me most: accurate news. During scans, focusing on my hope for accurate news helps me hold perfectly still. While awaiting results, that hope helps me prepare for any news.

When undergoing medical evaluations, the best news is accurate news—news that helps me move forward in healing ways.

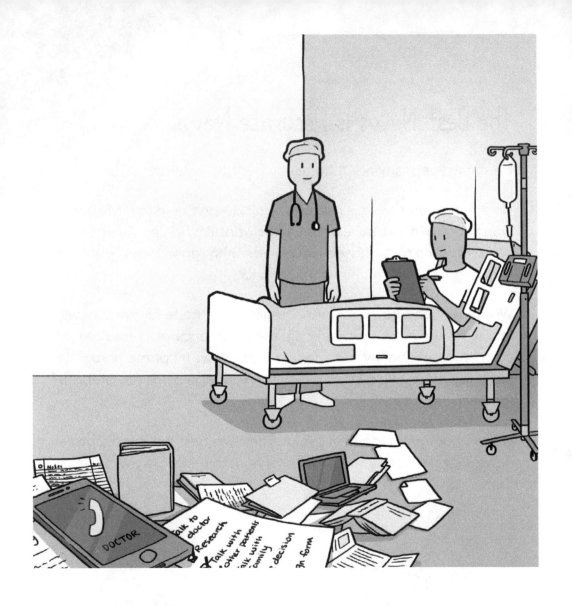

Informed Consent is a Process...
Not a Piece of Paper

Signing a consent form moments before elective surgery makes no sense. Who can think clearly while zoning out to keep from chickening out?

My solution: Delay scheduling any elective procedure until after my doctors have reviewed with me everything on the consent form and answered all my questions. Afterward, not rushed or frightened, I can make a fully informed decision. If I choose to proceed with surgery, then I can schedule it.

When the big day arrives, my signing the consent form simply affirms I haven't changed my mind. Without stress, my attention floats to hopeful, healing thoughts.

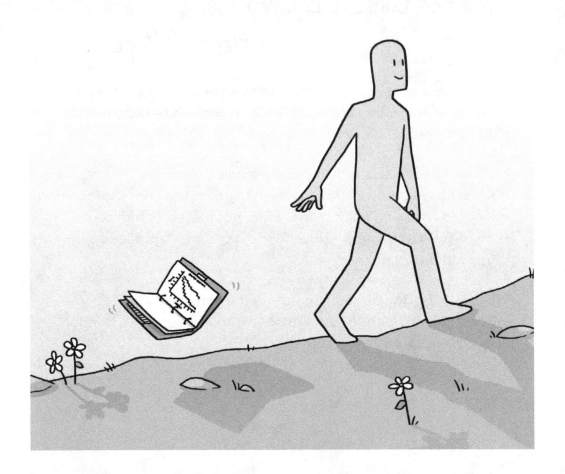

Statistics Don't Predict

Statistics about my disease sometimes make me feel hopeless. That's giving statistics too much power. I must always remember statistics are based on groups of past patients with similar cancers— and not on clones of "me" with my unique cancer.

Statistics help me get good care by guiding my doctors to the best treatment options. Statistics also help me live as fully as possible by preparing me for a likely course of events. But that's all. Statistics don't predict anything. I can always hope for the best possible outcome, no matter how unlikely.

After making my treatment decision, I have only this to say about unfavorable statistics:

> Statistics shmatistics.

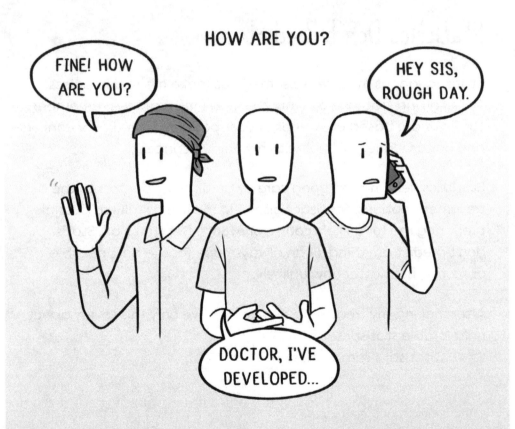

We Don't Need Scans to Know How We Are

A friend lovingly asks, "How are you?" I want to snap, "I'll find out after my next scans."

Before cancer, I always answered "How are you?" without hesitation. Back then, I didn't need to know what the coming week might bring. My answer depended on what I wanted or needed to share.

Why should now be any different? I know how I feel at the moment. I can usually tell what I want or need to share.

I don't need blood tests or scans to know how I am. I can continue to answer "How are you?" whichever way works for me.

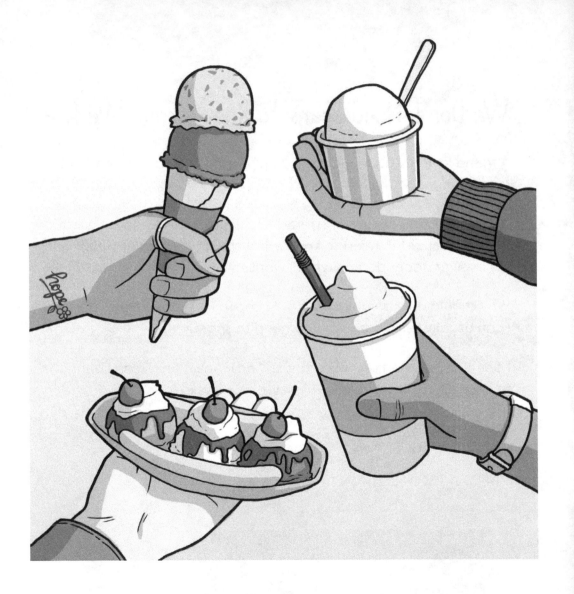

Everybody is Different...
Every Body is Different

Experts tell me what to expect at each stage of my survivorship. Other people's stories color my expectations with hopes and fears.

When talking with patients receiving similar treatments as me, I pay attention to every detail of stories that calm my fears and stoke my courage. I store those facts and images in the front of my mind, set to replay in tough times.

As for horror stories of medical complications and poor outcomes, I quickly label them "Not My Story." To prevent others' misfortunes from pulling me down, I keep repeating: "Everybody is different... every body is different."

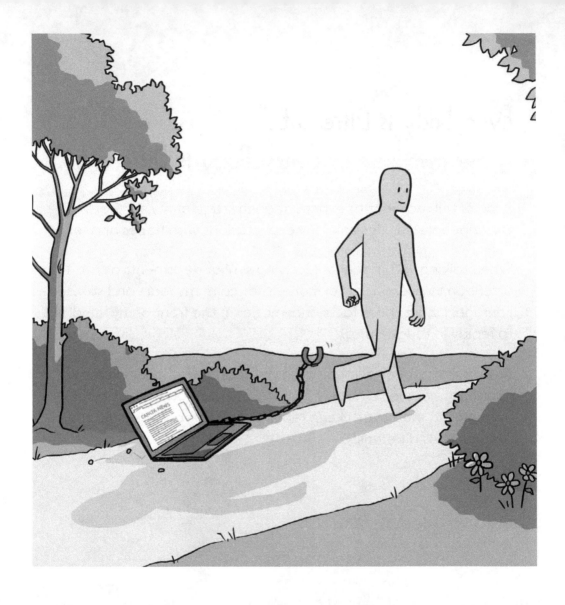

We Need to Know Enough, Not Everything

Some patients scour the internet every day for news about their type of cancer, even if they're doing well medically. Their ongoing research makes me uneasy.

Am I doing enough to stay healthy? Is it enough to eat a healthful diet, get some exercise, take my meds properly, go to checkups, and call my doctors about changes and problems?

Yes—as long as I don't need to make any medical decisions now. In times of stability, just knowing how to stay healthy is enough for me. I'd rather focus on things other than cancer.

Enough is enough.

Chapter 2:
Hope

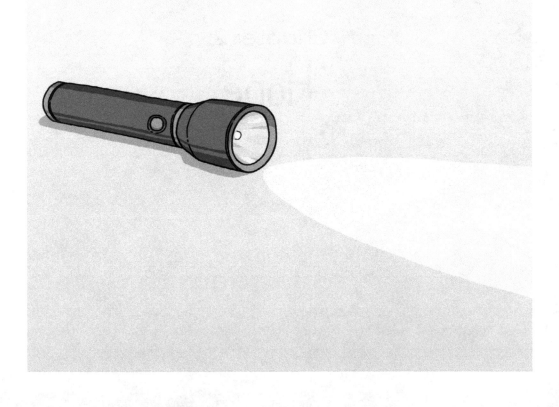

...about HOPE

Hope is a feeling linked to a belief. In particular, it's a pleasurable feeling that arises when we believe the desired outcome is possible for us. Our specific hopes lead us toward—or away from—Healthy Survivorship, depending on what we're hoping for.

Finding and nourishing healing hopes can be demanding work. It takes effort to distinguish helpful hopes from harmful hopes. It takes courage to let go (at least temporarily) of hopes that feel good but keep us from therapies or actions that help us in the long run. It takes strength to hold tightly to hopes that keep us whole.

May the affirmations in this chapter lead you to healing hopes— hopes that help you get good care and live as fully as possible.

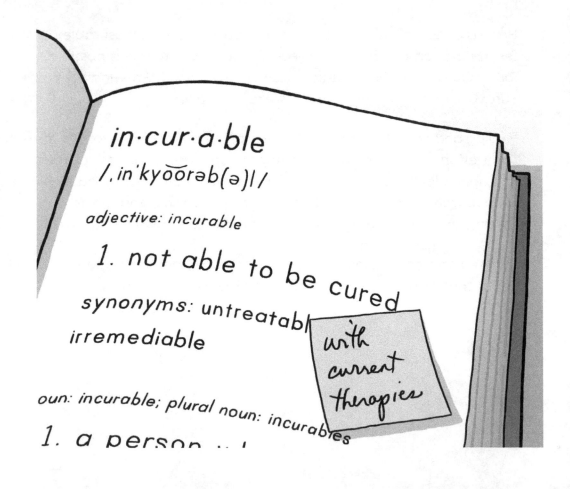

No Disease is Incurable

Some textbooks and doctors say, "That type of cancer is incurable." They're all wrong. They omitted the necessary concluding phrase: "with current therapies."

If other people describe their disease as incurable, I correct them in my head (and aloud, if appropriate) by adding the hopeful truth: "...with current therapies."

When talking about my own cancer, I confidently explain: "My cancer is treatable, with better treatments on the way. As long as there is research, my cancer is not incurable. It's a disease for which researchers are working toward a cure."

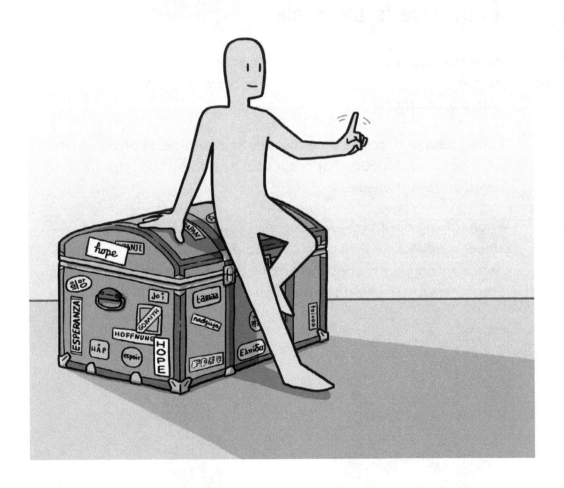

Doctors Can't Take Away Hope

If I ask my doctors, "Is there hope?" their answers reflect the statistical chance—the hope—of recovery. Their answer is not a statement about how much hope they feel or how much hope I should feel.

At every juncture, my physicians' job is to assess the most likely outcome and the best possible outcome for me. Since they can't predict the future, it's my job to decide which hopes to let go and which to continue holding tightly.

No doctors can take away my sense of hope, unless I let them. Like faith and love, hope arises within me. While there's life, I can always have hope of a better tomorrow.

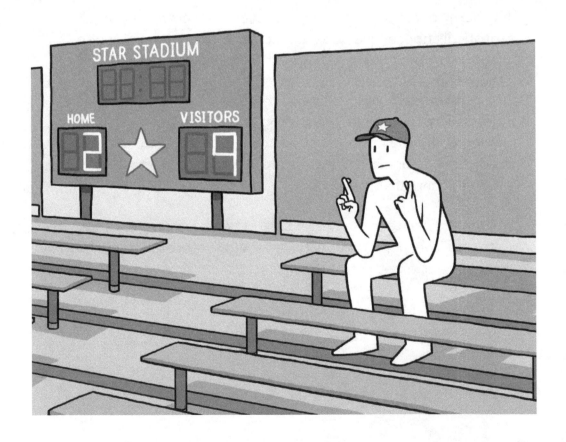

We Can Expect *That* and Hope *This*

Expectation and hope are two different things. I can expect one thing and, at the same time, hope for something else. If the odds are against my desired outcome, I can accept the sad news and expect the likely outcome while still hoping for the best possible outcome for me.

Decades ago I knew the statistics for my disease. I both expected to die from my cancer and hoped I'd be the long-lived outlier. Expectation helped me get things in order, in case. Hope helped me go through round after round of treatment.

Expectation is a state of mind that helps me prepare. Hope is a state of heart that helps me live.

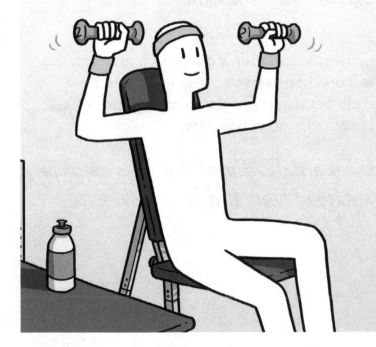

It's Best to Hope for the Best

When thinking about outcomes, the hope that helps me emotionally is hope for the best possible outcome. That hope helps me more than hope for a cure.

The best always feels within reach, because it is within reach.

Hope for the best mobilizes me to take health-promoting steps that improve my chance of the desired outcome, which increases my hopefulness even more, which decreases my stress and builds my confidence.

Nothing is better than best. That's why it's best to hope for the best. Hope for the best calms my anxiety about tomorrow and helps me live fully today.

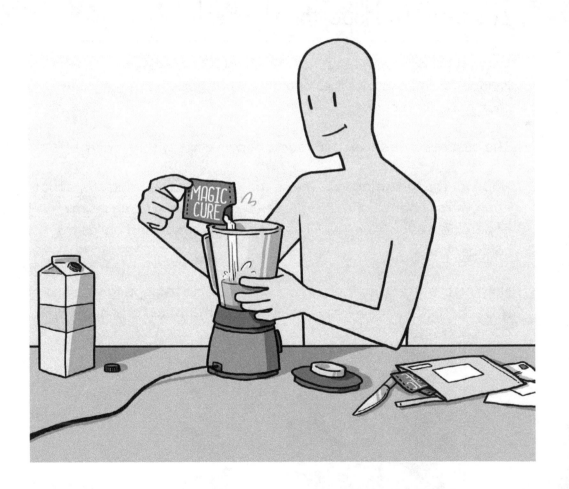

False Hope is a Real Feeling... that Disappoints

Someone offered me $1,000 to pick an ace from a deck of cards. Wanting the money, I dismissed the warnings of all the people who knew the four aces had been removed. While choosing a card I enjoyed the hope of winning, believing the deck was full and I had a real chance. What I was feeling was false hope—an uplifting feeling linked to a false premise.

False hope may comfort and inspire, just like realistic hope. But only for a while. Eventually, signs appear that the hoped-for goal won't be realized.

False hope is a real feeling that disappoints in the end. While making me feel good, false hope leads me away from Healthy Survivorship.

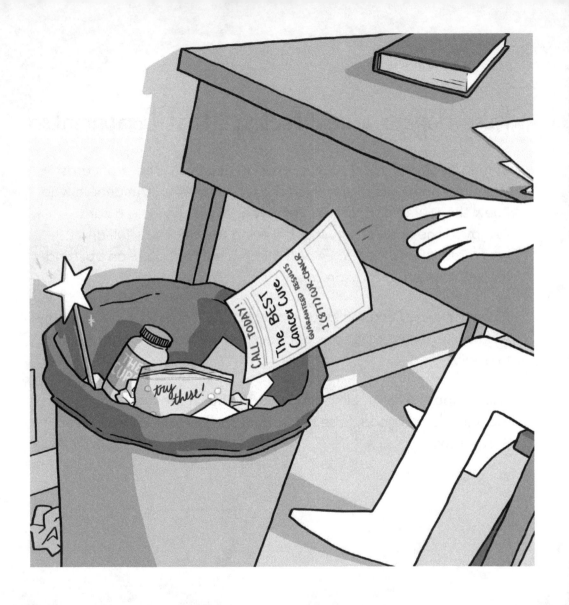

Avoiding Unrealistic Hope
Saves Time and Energy

When times are tough, it's tempting to hope for what I want—even if it sounds too good to be true. Unrealistic hopes, like wishes, help me feel better. Sadly, they don't help me get better.

Investing in unrealistic hopes wastes precious time and energy better directed toward realistic hopes—hopes that can be fulfilled.

Realistic hope drives me to decisions and actions that increase the chance—the hope—of the desired outcome. By improving my odds, I increase my sense of hope for a better tomorrow. Realistic hope is healing hope.

Realistic hope helps me feel better AND get better.

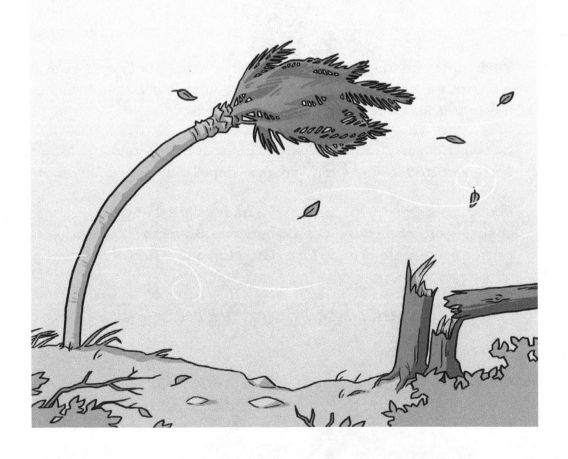

Reality-based Hope Waxes and Wanes

Sometimes I'm envious of patients who display unwavering hope. Their courage and confidence look so easy. I have to remind myself, "I'm not seeing their private moments."

If their hope is unwavering despite worrisome news, it's probably based on wishful thinking. Such rigid hope breaks when stressed.

Reality-based hope is flexible, which helps me adjust to setbacks. Since I'm not wasting emotional energy trying to deny known possibilities, I have more energy to hope for the best possible outcome for me.

Realistic hope waxes and wanes. Even at its lowest point, reality-based hope is more healing than hope based on wishful thinking.

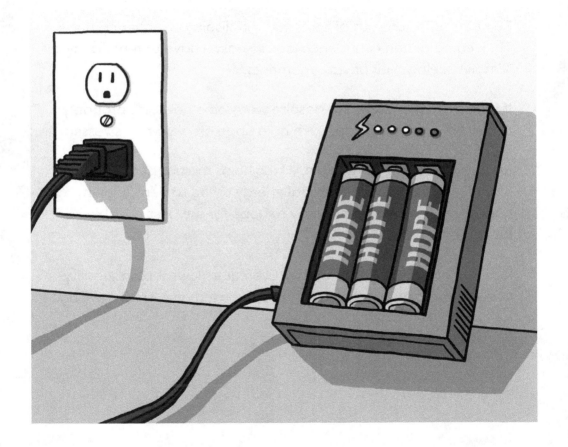

Hope Needs Recharging

Hope is a feeling. All feelings are fleeting. To keep my hope from fading away, every day I take steps to energize my hope. My favorite ways include...

- listening to others' success stories
- helping someone else
- reading inspirational sayings
- reciting uplifting prayers
- listening to lively music
- renewing a subscription

Recharging hope keeps hope strong.

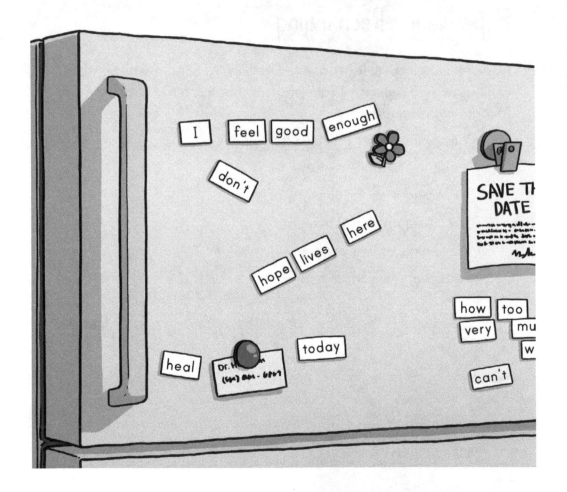

Hopeful Language Nurtures Hope

Minor word changes help me heal by turning expressions of despair into hopeful calls for understanding and patience.

"It's too painful" means I'm overwhelmed. By saying, "It's very painful," I'm describing my challenge, without any judgment about my ability to cope.

"I can't..." declares my inability to function, triggering grief. By saying "Right now, I can't...," I narrow the time frame of my debility and create space for hope. Similarly, tacking on "yet"—as in, "I can't... yet"—transforms expressions of loss into testaments of hope.

Whenever talking about my challenges, I nourish hope by speaking in the language of hope.

Hope spoken here.

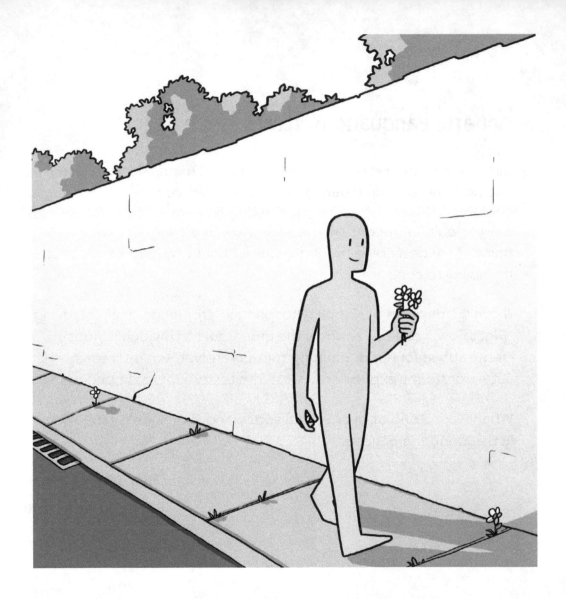

If There is Hope, We Have Reason to Hope

In times of uncertainty, there's always hope of the best outcome. Here, "hope" means "possibility." That's different than having hope, where "hope" is a feeling. As long as there is hope (as in, possibility) of the desired outcome, I have reason to have the feeling of hope.

Cicero teaches, "While there's life, there's hope." Whatever my situation, I can always have hope for something good. For example, I can hope to make wise treatment decisions; to treat my disease while better therapies are being developed; to avoid futile treatments; and to create a legacy of meaningful moments. I can always hope for recovery or a longer time than expected.

Where there is hope, there is life.

Chapter 3:
Action

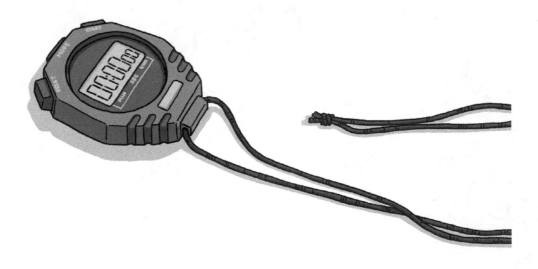

...about ACTION

If the squeak of a rusty hinge hurts our ears every time we open a door, knowing how to fix it and hoping to fix it are only a start. To obtain relief from the painful noise, we must act and squirt oil on the offending hinge.

Similarly, Healthy Survivorship depends on taking actions that help us heal. As patients, taking proper action can be challenging. We often need to overcome practical and emotional obstacles to acting on our knowledge and hope in healthy ways.

May these affirmations help you find the courage, motivation, patience and fortitude needed to narrow the gap between knowing what to do and taking action to do it.

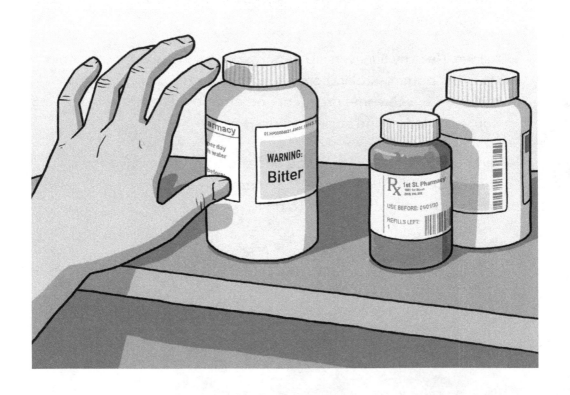

Worst First Works Best

Some health-promoting measures are uncomfortable, inconvenient or tedious. Naturally, those are the ones I tend to delay acting on. Here's the problem: Choosing to delay is choosing to lose the benefits of proper action.

One solution is to do the dreaded tasks first, while I'm fresh. Tackling the worst first minimizes my anticipatory distress and maximizes my chance of success.

If an unpleasant task threatens my day, I gear up quickly and don't delay. Then I'm over the worst and free to play, knowing I gave it my best.

Worst first.

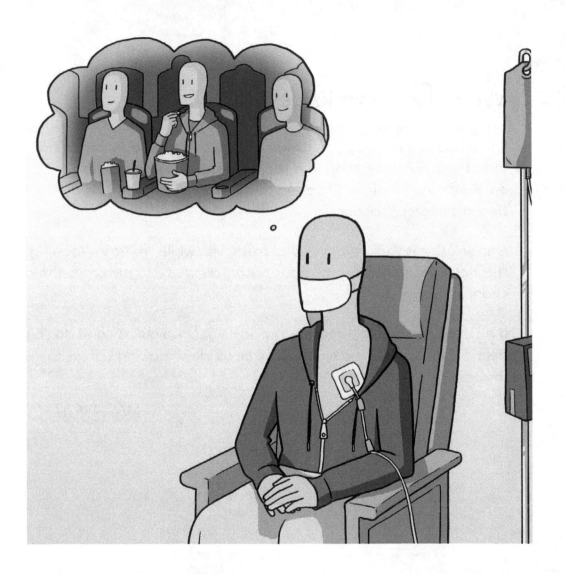

Thinking About Tomorrow Helps Us Act Today

"Live in the moment." That wise adage for enjoying life to the fullest can become an obstacle to taking proper action.

While tackling unpleasant tasks of Healthy Survivorship, the notion of living in the moment focuses my attention on my pain or loss. That exacerbates my negative emotions, which makes it tough to follow through.

If the task is challenging, I can proceed with proper action more easily by envisioning all the ways I'll benefit in the future. I can anticipate feeling satisfied when the task is behind me, knowing I've done my best.

In the face of hardship, I don't always live in the moment. At times, thinking about tomorrow helps me take proper action today.

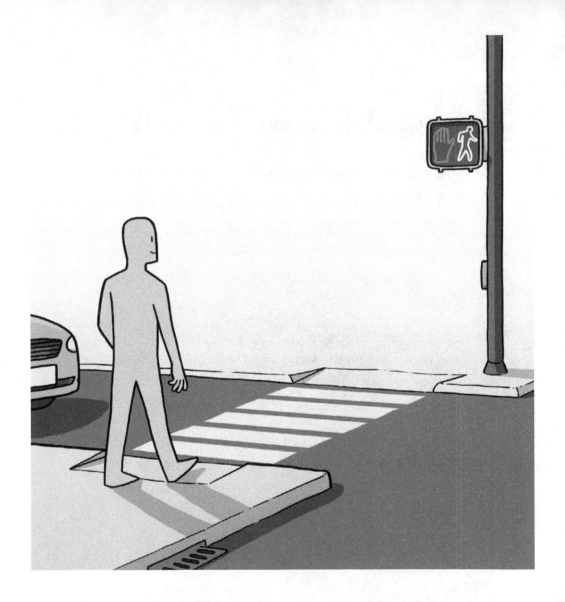

Rules Are Our Friends

I realize my doctors' rules are intended to protect me. Yet I don't like how their rules—You can't do this. You must do that—make me feel powerless and constrained.

Here's my 2-step trick for maintaining a sense of control if instincts or desires tempt me to break a rule "just this once." First, I imagine facing the problem the rule was designed to prevent. Then I ask myself, "Was the benefit of breaking the rule worth having to deal with this problem now?"

Rules put me in control by making it easier to decide what to do. Rules empower me to take the best action when emotions tempt me otherwise. Rules keep me in control by preventing problems.

Rules are my friends — but only if I respect them.

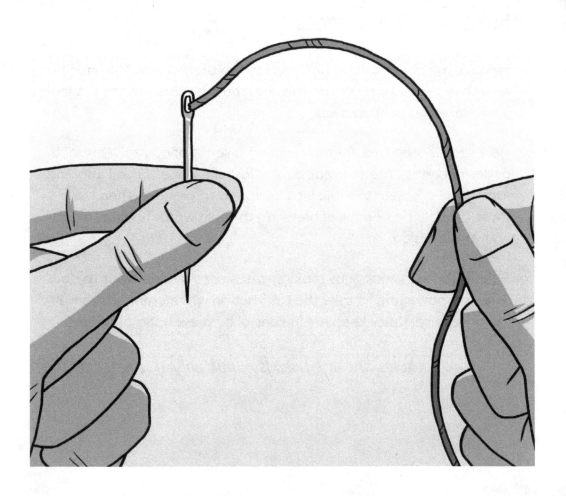

If It Were Easy to Do, It Would Be Easy to Do

Sometimes I know what to do, yet mess up. That means only one thing: The task was challenging in some way.

By exploring what might have tripped me up, I can brainstorm various ways to overcome the obstacles. Refining my approach to the challenge should make it easier to do next time. Through trial and error, I'll keep refining my approach until I succeed most times, if not every time.

Of course, some tasks never get easy. I can succeed at those tasks, too, especially if expecting difficult tasks to be difficult to do.

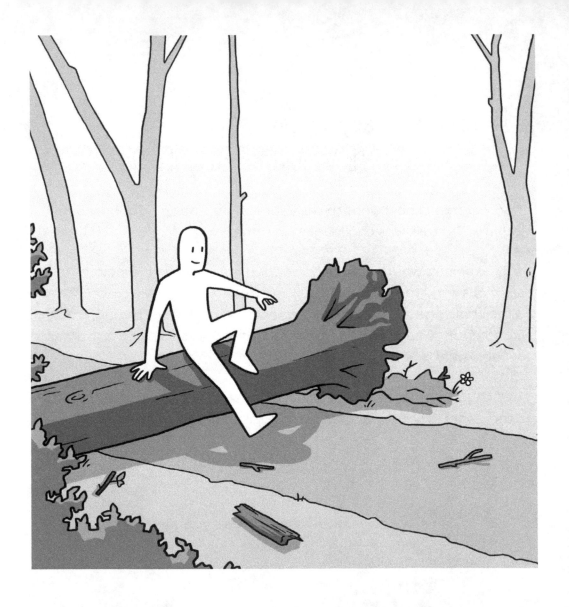

Our Best is the Best We Can Do

When I suffer a setback, it does not mean I did anything wrong. It means something we knew could happen did happen.

It's like the time I wisely picked the shortest checkout line. Then, one customer ahead of me needed a price check and another paid in pennies. I ended up waiting longer than had I picked another line. My choice was still wise; it just didn't work out.

In any situation where the outcome is affected by factors beyond my control or ability to predict, I cannot possibly know the "right" choice ahead of time.

The best I can do is the best I can do.
And the best is good enough.

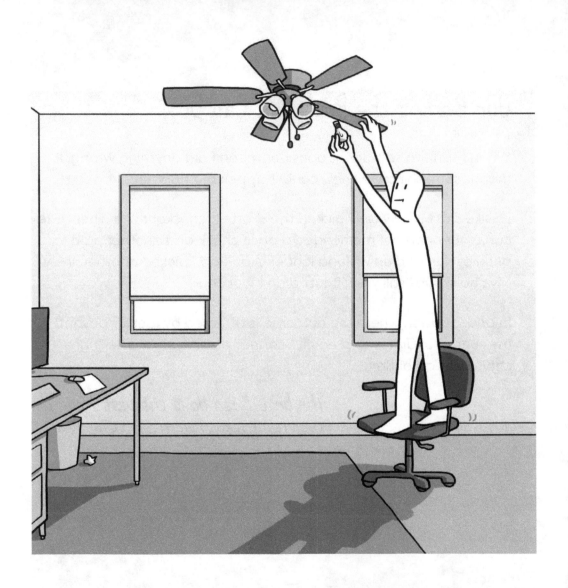

Illness Makes Smart People Do Foolish Things

I've done a few foolish things while dealing with my health. Knowing the best thing to do, I did something else that was easier or more appealing in some way. I'm not alone.

Plenty of people who know better do foolish things on occasion, such as keep secret a new symptom or delay needed tests and treatments. Nobody's perfect.

When I don't take proper action, I forgive myself for being human—but do not excuse my action. I use the episode positively by renewing my commitment to act on my knowledge and hope in healthy ways.

If I'm tempted to take needless risks or miss opportunities to make things better, I encourage myself: Don't be foolish. Do what's best.

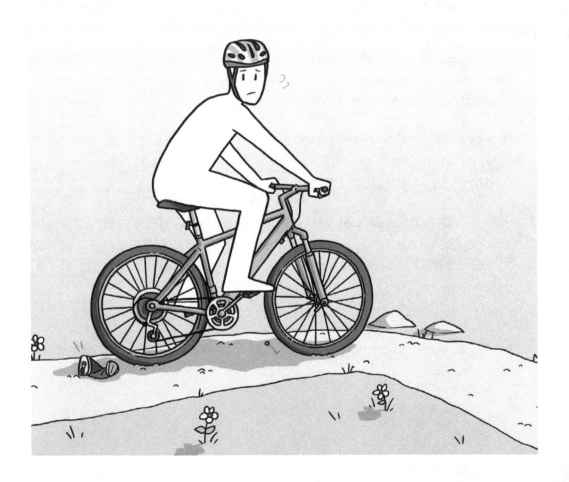

Face Forward to Move Forward

Missteps happen. The problem to avoid is ruminating over a slip-up. I need to keep looking forward. Looking back distracts me from the challenges in front of me, putting me at risk of missteps and missed opportunities for improvement.

It's healthy to reflect briefly on what went wrong in the past. Doing so enables me to find ways to put closure on it and avoid a similar problem in the future.

It's not healing to linger on my regret, anger, disappointment or embarrassment about something in the past. Letting go of yesterday and facing forward enables me to see—and take—my best path to tomorrow.

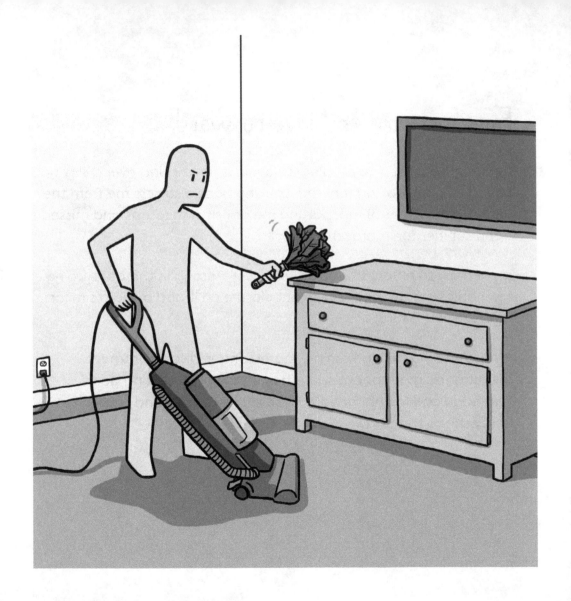

Negative Energy Can Fuel Positive Action

If negative emotions bog me down, I remind myself that energy is energy. The negative energy of fear, anger and frustration can galvanize me in productive ways, just as the positive energy of hope, confidence and gratitude motivates me to get jobs done.

That's why I no longer dread scanxiety—anxiety about forthcoming scans. With cancer testing a regular part of my life, I can regularly channel that extra squirt of energy into making progress on projects I want or need to get done.

Whenever I can, I use negative energy to fuel positive action.

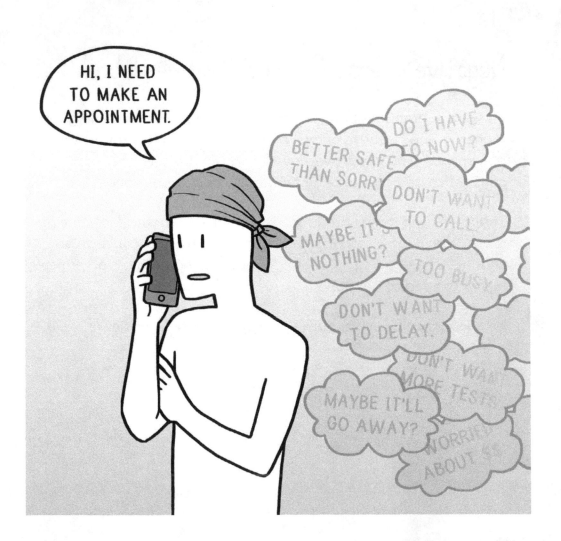

Action is the Final Answer

To benefit from health-promoting measures, the only thing that matters is whether I take proper action. In most cases, it doesn't matter if I take action easily and independently, or with difficulty and lots of assistance, or anything in-between.

For example, I promote healing by eating a healthy diet. My cells don't know if I enjoy cooking or hate being in the kitchen. Or if I enjoy organic fruits and vegetables or prefer junk food. Or if I made the meals myself or paid someone to prepare them. All that matters is which nutrients reach the cells in my body.

When it comes to making things better, action is the final answer.

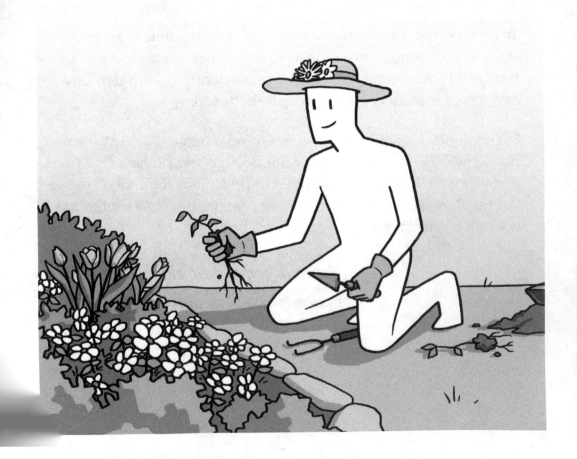

Healthy Survivorship is Always a Work-In-Progress

Healthy Survivorship is hard work. Every day, obstacles get in the way of obtaining good care or living as fully as possible. Stubborn old obstacles. New ones as I change or as my circumstances change.

The pursuit of Healthy Survivorship is like climbing a never-ending staircase. Each time I take proper action, I've strengthened my muscles for that action. And like after taking a step up, I now enjoy a wider view that helps me next time. If improper action causes me to slip down a step or two, I can learn something useful for increasing the chance of success next time.

Whether steadily climbing up or taking two-steps-up-one-step-down, proper action is always a work-in-progress. And that's okay.

Chapter 4:
Meaning

...about MEANING

The aphorisms in this chapter address issues of meaning. What do our test results mean? What does it mean if we say we're tired and friends respond by telling us they're tired too? What is the meaning of our illness?

Disease affects only our body. However the illness—the thoughts, feelings, stresses, losses and pain—affects every fiber of our being. Reflecting on issues of meaning opens the possibility of benefiting from reordered life priorities, a new sense of self, and a transformed vision of what it means to triumph in life.

May the aphorisms in this chapter give new meaning to your challenges, meaning that helps you embrace life in healing ways.

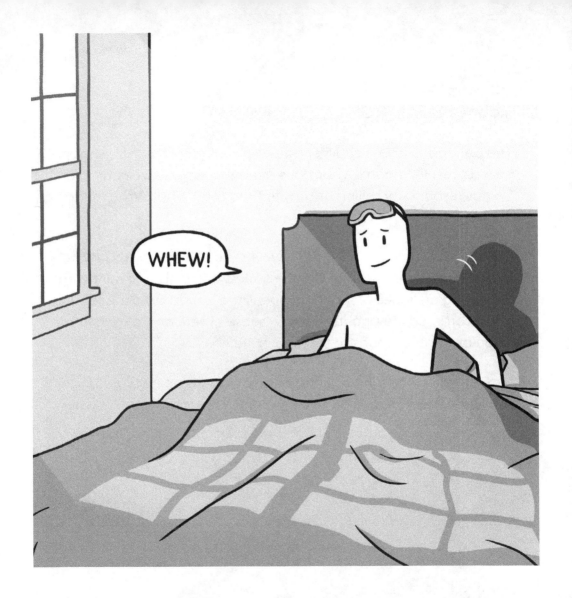

Dreams Are Imaginary... Not Reality

My hammering heart awakens me from a nightmare about a health disaster. Is my dream a sign? No. Most likely, my brain cells simply misfired. Awash in chemicals released by stress, fatigue and medications, my brain conjured images that, like carnival mirrors, distorted reality in meaningless ways.

Maybe the dream was my body's way of responding to suppressed fears or anxieties. Maybe not. Either way, nightmares can be used for healing if they motivate me to talk about feelings that bother me during the day and, if needed, to get help dealing with them. Nightmares are healing if they scare me into taking proper action while I'm awake.

Dreams don't predict the future.

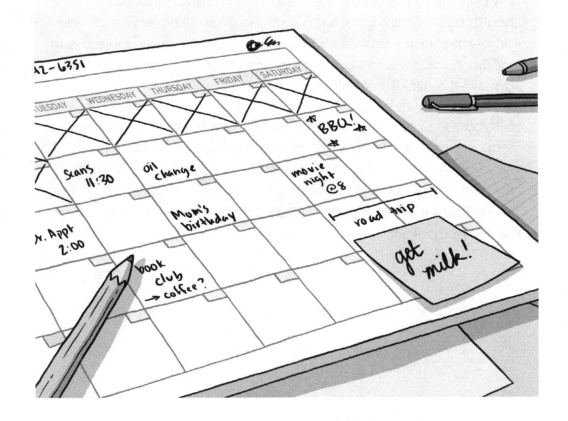

Cancer Doesn't Make Life Uncertain

After my cancer diagnosis, life felt distressingly uncertain. I agonized over whether to renew my magazine subscriptions. Party invitations sent me into a tizzy: Should I accept, not knowing if I'll feel well enough to go?

Before my diagnosis I'd accepted invitations, knowing I could end up cancelling due to, say, car trouble or the flu. Years later, I attended the funeral of someone who had no health issues when I was first sick and had talked confidently of his long-term plans.

Cancer doesn't make life uncertain. Cancer simply exposes the uncertainty of life. Cancer makes life feel more uncertain. I'll keep planning for tomorrow while living fully today.

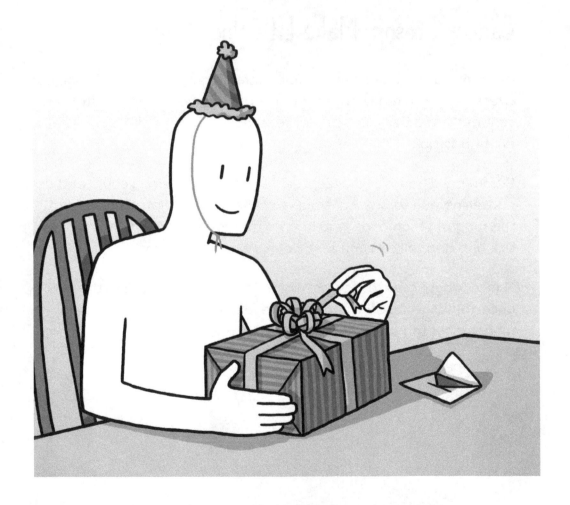

A Certain Uncertainty is a Wonderful Thing

My friend is thrilled to learn my cancer is in remission. "Don't you wish you knew if you were cured?" I immediately respond, "No!" Perplexed, she asks why not.

I explain there are only two ways to know if I'm cured. If my cancer recurs, I'll know I am not cured. If my cancer is in remission when I'm dying of something else, I'll know I am cured. So, no, I don't want to know if I'm cured.

To live fully today, I don't need to know if I'm cured. I don't want to know, either. After cancer, a certain uncertainty is a wonderful thing.

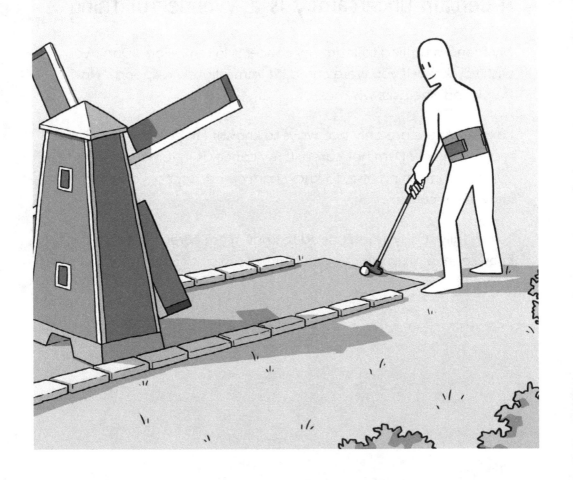

Feeling Good Enough is Good Enough

When friends and family ask me how I'm feeling, I don't like to lie. Here's my problem: While in treatment, I don't like talking about the side effects that make me feel under par. While in remission, I don't like talking about the aftereffects that prevent me from feeling great.

One day, someone asked the usual, "How are you feeling?" I surprised myself by blurting out, "Good enough!" It was true. I felt well enough to be doing what I was doing (otherwise I wouldn't have been doing it, right?).

When it comes to living well after cancer, I don't need to feel completely well to have a great day or to love my life. "Good enough" is good enough for me.

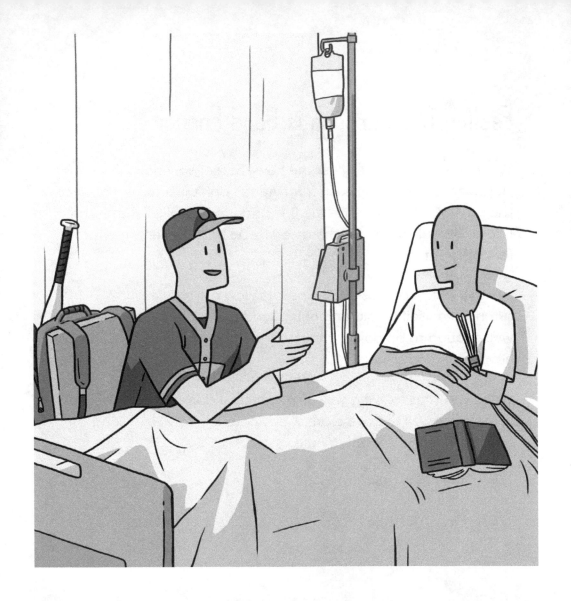

We Don't Need Everyone to Understand

"I'm tired and feel so vulnerable," I'd say. Friends would respond, "I'm tired, too. And I could get hit by a bus on my way home." Their well-intended efforts to normalize my experience made me feel isolated. I wished they understood.

It's human nature to want others to understand. Life became easier after I realized I don't need casual friends and coworkers to understand what I am experiencing, as long as they are not hurting me.

As for close family and friends, I still wish they understood. That's asking a lot, though, if they've never been through something similar. With loved ones, I don't need them to understand—as long as they believe me and care.

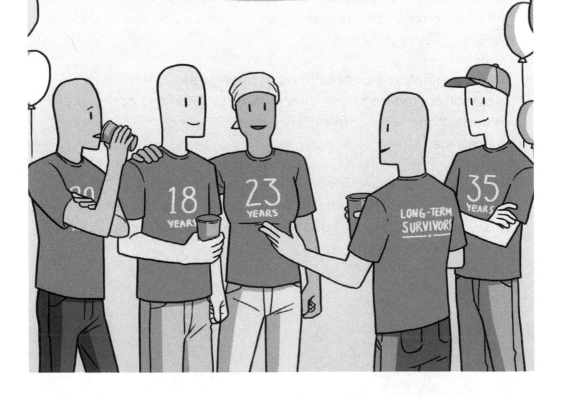

Worry About Late Effects is a Luxury

My cancer treatments put me at risk of late effects, namely problems that develop long after completion of treatment. I'm at peace regarding that risk. Why?

For one thing, I know most long-term survivors don't develop serious late effects. For another, I can minimize the chance of developing some of the serious problems by following a healthy lifestyle and by reporting worrisome symptoms.

The biggest reason I don't worry much about late effects is because I remember a time when my long-term prognosis was poor. Back then, I envied patients whose prognosis was good enough to make late effects an issue. Worry about late effects is a luxury reserved for patients with a good prognosis and for long-term survivors.

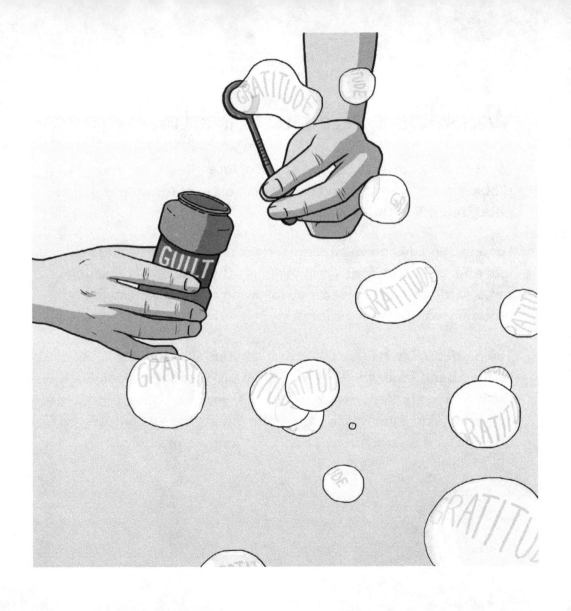

We Honor Others By Turning Survivor's Guilt into Gratitude

Survivor's guilt. That's what people call the uneasiness I feel when friends with cancer die. It's a misnomer. Why should I feel guilty? I haven't done anything wrong. My survival doesn't hurt anyone else's chance of survival. Surviving has nothing to do with deserving to live and everything to do with treatment working.

My uneasiness is not guilt. There's no word for this mix of empathy for others, grief stirred by imagining what I might have lost, and a twinge of shame that I'm relieved it wasn't me.

I honor those who died by choosing to use this uncomfortable feeling to motivate me to feel heightened gratitude for all that is good in my world.

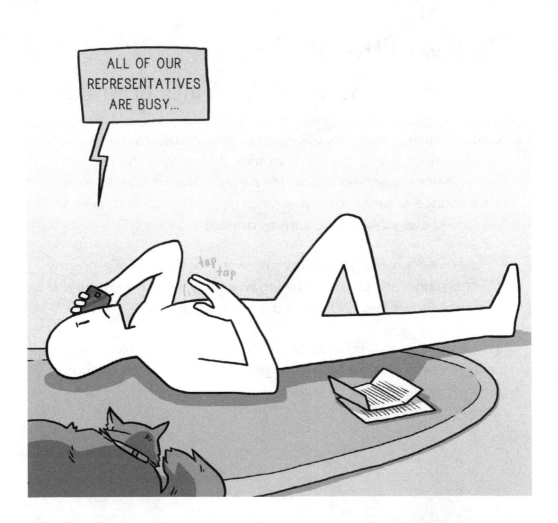

Unpleasant Times Prove We Are Here

Life is full of challenges. While dealing with the stresses of illness and recovery, the mundane hassles of everyday life can feel burdensome. Crises can feel overwhelming.

If I'm worn out when problems arise, one option is to let others take over. Delegating does not mean I'm weak or shirking responsibilities. It means I'm prioritizing wisely to preserve my well-being.

Other times, I want to handle a problem myself, even though others could take over. Or it's a life problem that only I can address. In those cases, I dig deep and give it my best.

Life is not easy for anyone. Whether I am delegating or digging deep, I now find unpleasant times less painful because they are proof that I am still here.

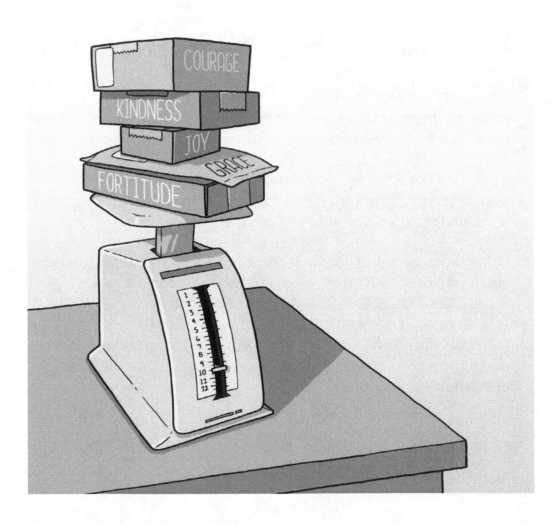

Triumph Over Cancer is Measured
by How We Live

What does it mean to triumph over cancer? Most people assume it means being cured or, at least, living a long, long time. That view misses the point of life.

I've seen people cured of disease but living in an emotional web of poor self-esteem, fear of recurrence, and bitterness about their losses. They've survived, but not triumphed.

I've also seen—and admired—people who experienced meaningful moments and created joyful memories in whatever time they had. They triumphed, whether they survived 10 years or 10 months.

Triumph over cancer is measured by how I live—not how long.

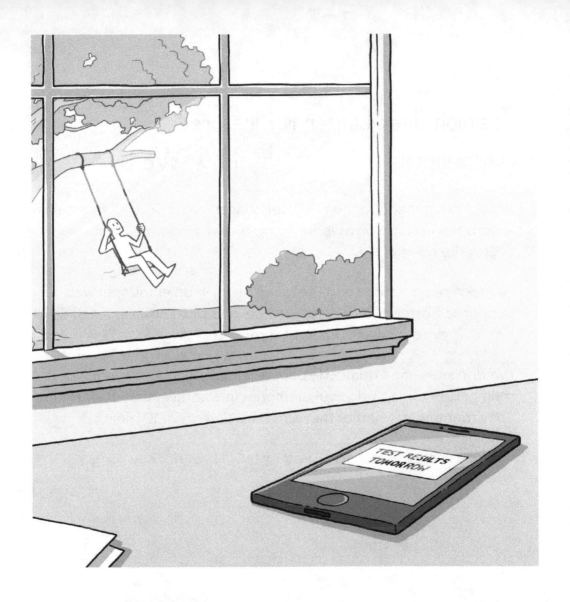

Don't Wait and See... Live and See

Being a patient involves lots of waiting. Waiting for appointments. Waiting for test results. Waiting for symptoms to resolve. Waiting to see how things will turn out. If I focus on the waiting while in the limbo of Wait-and-See, soon I'll be living in the land of Worry-and-See—and that is not a good way to live.

I have too much living to do today to put my life on hold while waiting to find out what will happen tomorrow. Never again will I wait and see.

I have today. While waiting for news or anything else, I'll live and see.

Chapter 5:
Happiness

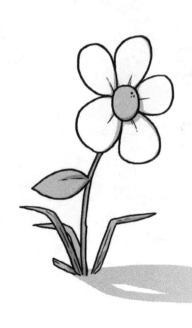

...about HAPPINESS

What's the point of surviving if we don't enjoy our life? After cancer, happiness can feel elusive. Pain, fatigue and medications, as well as fear, grief and other unpleasant emotions, can make happiness seem impossible. It's not.

After cancer we can expect to find some happiness. At times, we may have to work with our healthcare team to overcome medical obstacles to happiness. We often have to invest time and energy in efforts that set the stage for happiness.

May these aphorisms help you find some happiness despite illness and tap into the special happiness that occasionally happens because of illness.

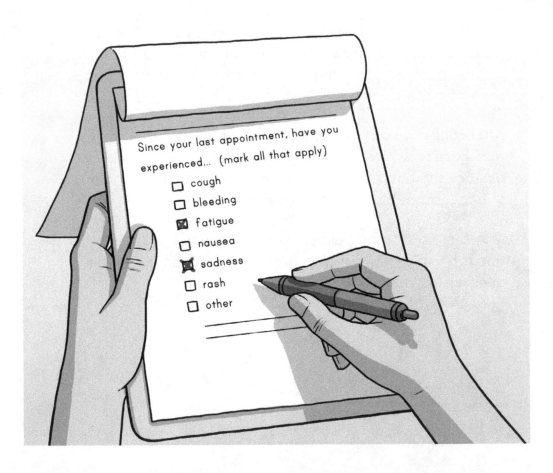

Unhappiness is a Symptom

I can't feel happy while someone is smashing my toes with a hammer. Similarly, medical conditions can interfere with the pathways in my brain that give rise to the feeling of joy.

That's why I report unhappiness to my doctors the same way I report bleeding or a cough. Together, we can address medical issues that may be playing a role, such as pain, sleep deprivation, certain medications, malnutrition, grief or chronic stress.

Unhappiness deserves the same medical attention as a cough. Fixing problems that interfere with happiness is good for my health and good for my life.

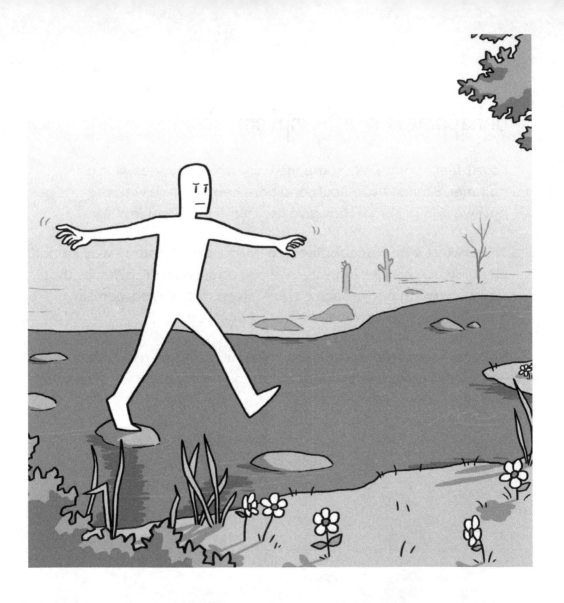

Transitions are Trying... and Temporary

I expected to feel blue while my hair was falling out and while sick and tired from chemo. The surprise came while celebrating my remission. Unhappiness blindsided me. Why now?

Transitions—including happy ones—involve new routines, roles and rules. New worries can arise, such as the fear of recurrence that first revs up after treatment ends. New losses may be realized, including those due to changes that happened months ago but had no impact until now.

Transitions are trying. Expecting difficulties helps.

Transitions are also temporary. Adjusting to the changes and losses paves the way to new happiness.

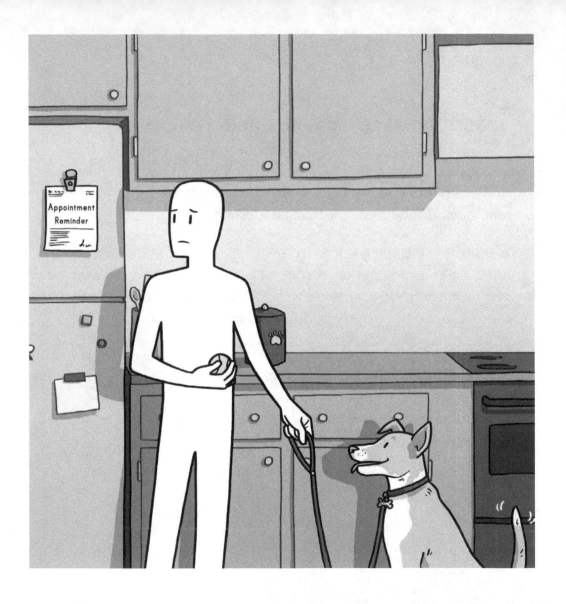

Fear Tomorrow; Miss Today

I heard of a woman who was doing well after completing her cancer treatment. Yet she began each day thinking,

"Today might be the day my cancer comes back."

Her fear of recurrence led her to withdraw from activities and relationships that used to bring her joy. Night after night she went to bed after a long empty day.

A year passed. Two, three... seven years went by. Then her fear became reality. She was devastated by her recurrence.

"I was well all that time," she cried. "And I missed it."

That true story convinced me I had to learn to calm my fears of tomorrow, so I could enjoy today. I have today. I refuse to miss it.

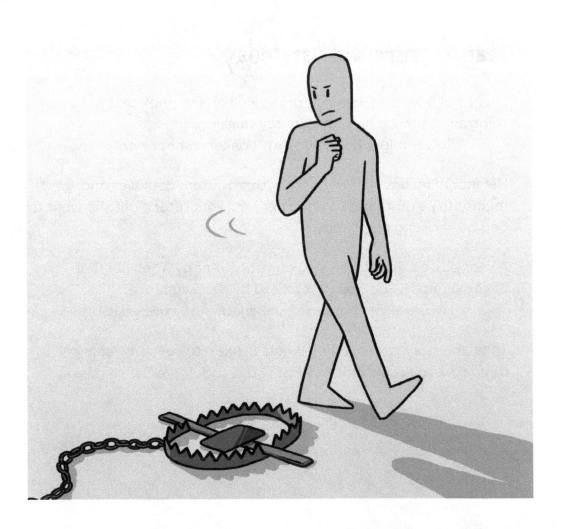

Hassles are Just Gumption Traps

What do a flat tire and a snafu with my blood test have in common? They're both gumption traps, hassles that deplete my initiative and resolve—my gumption.

Gumption traps threaten to leave me discouraged, agitated, sad and/or angry. Without my gumption, my outlook may turn little problems into existential issues of "Why me?" Happiness becomes almost impossible.

If a hassle threatens to drain my gumption, I put a stop to it. How? By calling the problem "a gumption trap," and not "a crisis." I see the hassle as an annoying chore for my to-do list—and nothing more.

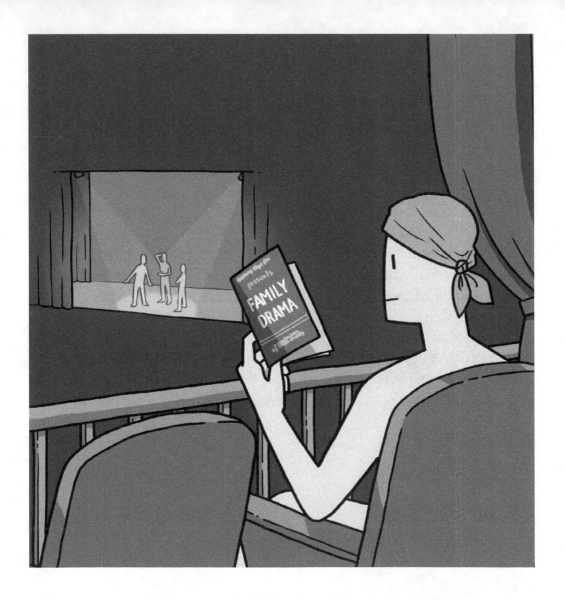

Sometimes the Best Seat is in the Balcony

Others' news affects me. If my own happiness feels fragile, thinking about others' problems can tip me over. Creating emotional distance from others' woes helps preserve my happiness.

If watching TV coverage of a disaster, I change the channel, knowing I still care. If a friend is bereaved, I send a heartfelt note and let others provide the in-person support I'd usually offer. If a loved one is dealing with ongoing family problems, I imagine climbing to the back row of the balcony to watch their drama from afar.

If I'm not needed to fix a problem, the best thing I can do for everyone is to take a seat in the balcony. Preserving my emotional reserves helps me heal today, so I can be there for others tomorrow.

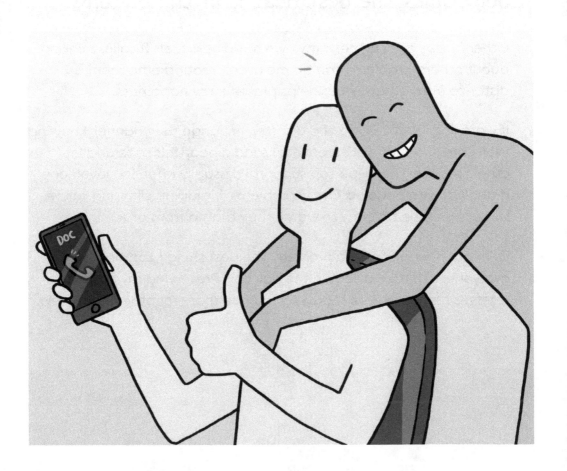

False Alarms are Reasons to Celebrate

Hallelujah! My worrisome symptom turned out to be nothing. Why don't I feel happy? Instead, I feel embarrassed about sounding the alarm. I feel guilty about wasting my doctors' time and unnecessarily worrying my loved ones.

I shouldn't. I did the right thing to report my symptom. My doctors did the right thing to evaluate it because the symptom may have signaled a problem needing medical attention.

False alarms are part of survivorship. Lucky for me, we got the results I wanted, and not the results I feared.

False alarms give me reasons to celebrate. I can stop wondering and worrying what the symptom means. I don't have to deal with new treatments. Yay, I'm okay.

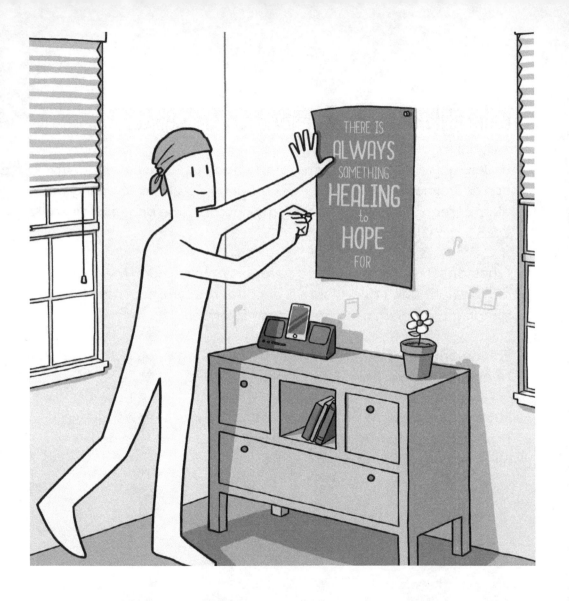

We Can Always Set the Stage for Happiness

A popular refrigerator magnet suggests all I need to do to feel happy is "Choose Happiness!" Sadly, it's not true. Here's the good news: I can always choose to set the stage for happiness.

How? I can create a space where I am surrounded by sights, scents and sounds that please me: Pictures of loved ones and happy memories; favorite candles and lotions; inspirational sayings; music; clothes in my favorite colors and fabrics. I can put myself in situations that usually bring joy, such as doing a favorite activity or being with favorite people.

Whatever the circumstances, I can set the stage for happiness.

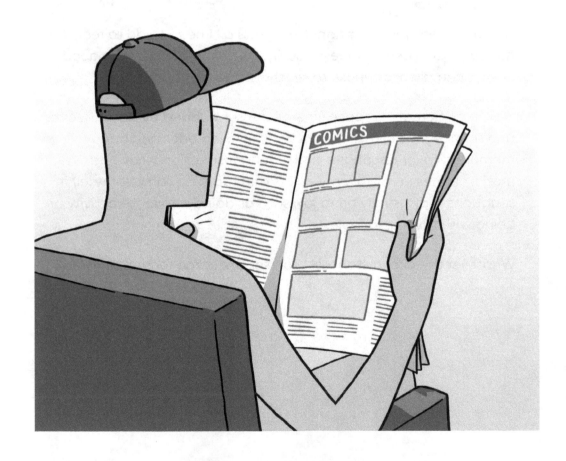

Cancer Humor is Good Medicine

Cancer is never funny. That said, cancer sometimes puts me in situations that are amusing, if I'm willing to look for the humor in tough times.

Age-old wisdom dictates that laughter is healing medicine. By joking about problems, such as my hair loss or my genetic mutation, I regain a sense of power over things that sadden or frighten me. Joking about illness can help strengthen my hope of recovery. Besides, when I'm laughing I can't be crying, which is nice.

To keep sadness at bay, at least once a day I look for ways to tickle my funny bone.

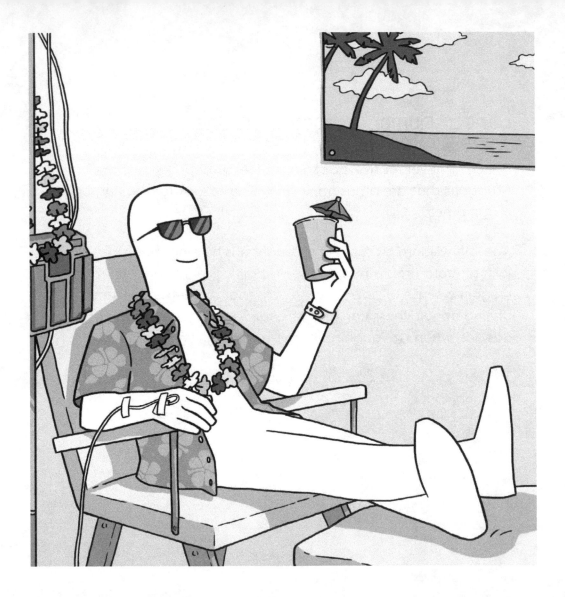

Regular Mini-Holidays Help Us Heal

Holidays are festive breaks from my routine. When I need a break from cancer, I create a mini-holiday. For a day or even just one hour, I find or create a space that feels far from the demands and stresses of cancer.

My oasis can be any activity that follows one rule: No thinking or talking about cancer. Sometimes I escape to a comfy chair and listen to my iPod or indulge in a favorite movie. Other times I take a walk or enjoy a phone visit with a friend or loved one, keeping to our rule: No cancer talk.

I don't need a national holiday to enjoy a festive break. I just need to create a joyful space and go there.

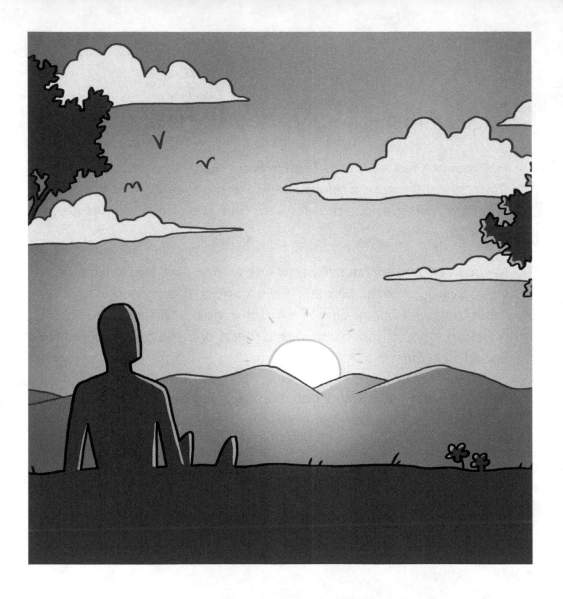

Celebrating Today Acknowledges All That is Good

I'm not yet out of the woods. Some people think it's not time to celebrate. I disagree. It's precisely because tomorrow is uncertain that celebrating today makes all the sense in the world.

Cake and balloons. High fives and hugs. These things create sensory feasts that enhance joyful feelings about an accomplishment or anniversary. Celebrating ordinary pleasures acknowledges all that is right in my world. In good times, celebrations keep me grateful. In tough times, celebrations keep me hopeful. Sometimes the only thing to celebrate is that I made it through today.

Every day the choice is mine: How shall I celebrate today?

Epilogue

Since my diagnosis in 1990, I've strived to get good care and live as fully as possible—in other words, to be a Healthy Survivor. Every step of the way I have needed hope. Over the years of trial-and-error, I've gotten better and better at figuring out what to hope for each day and how to nourish healing hopes. I'm still learning.

I hope the insights shared in this book help you think in new ways about hope and help you find healing hopes for you. I hope some of the aphorisms work well for you, either as is or after you edit them to work well for your personal circumstances. I hope your self-talk helps you tap into your inner courage, fortitude, patience and confidence. I hope you see and enjoy whatever happiness is possible in whatever time you have.

My greatest hope is for you, too, to become a Healthy Survivor.

Hope

Hope is an image of goals planted firmly in your mind.
When looking at life before you, hope lines the paths you find.

Hope is a well of courage nestled deep within your heart.
When faltering in fear and doubt, hope pushes you to start.

Hope is an urge to keep going, for limbs too tired and weak.
When apathy stills all desire, hope sparks the fuel you seek.

Hope is a promise of patience as you wait for distress to wane.
When all you can do is nothing, hope pulls you through the pain.

Hope is a spirit that lifts you, should heaviness pull at your soul.
When torn apart by losses, hope mends to keep you whole.

[from, *Happiness in a Storm*]

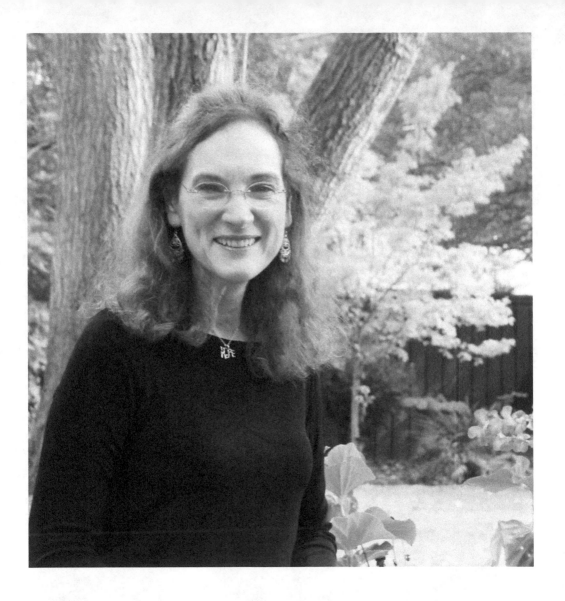

About the Author

Wendy S. Harpham was a solo practitioner of internal medicine when diagnosed with non-Hodgkin's lymphoma in 1990. Forced by ongoing illness to retire from clinical medicine in 1993, Dr. Harpham turned to writing and speaking to continue to educate, comfort and inspire patients.

In addition to her books, Harpham writes a popular column for clinicians in *Oncology Times*, titled "View from the Other Side of the Stethoscope," and a blog on Healthy Survivorship. She travels coast to coast and internationally, delivering keynotes to professional and lay audiences. Her work has been honored with numerous awards, including the Governor's Award for Health, for which she was inducted into the Texas Women's Hall of Fame.

Dr. Harpham advocates for patients through her participation in local and national working groups and patient advisory councils. She is an adjunct professor at the University of Texas at Dallas, where she co-teaches an honors seminar, offers writing workshops, and mentors premedical students.

She lives in Dallas with her husband, a professor of political philosophy, and enjoys frequent visits with her three Dallas-based children and their families.

About the Illustrator

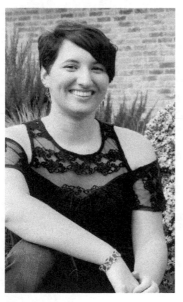

Family lore includes Emma learning to use a crayon before she learned to use a spoon. Growing up, her insatiable passion for the visual arts took her to art camps and programs, including the Charleston County School of the Arts.

Since 2014, Emma has been an honors student and National Merit Scholar at the University of Texas at Dallas. In May 2018, she will graduate with a Bachelor of Arts from the School of Arts, Technology, and Emerging Communication.

From the day Emma learned of this project, she embraced the mission of helping patients get good care and live as fully as possible. The art and design of *Healing Hope* marks her professional debut as an illustrator. For more, visit *emmathes.com*.

9 780999 708811